NATURAL JOINT PAIN REMEDY

Effective Home Remedies for Managing Joint Pain Naturally

e Kelly

Copyright

Table of Contents

Chapter 1:
Understanding Joint Pain: Causes and Symptoms

Joint pain is a common health issue that affects millions of people worldwide. It can be caused by a variety of factors and can have a significant impact on quality of life. In this chapter, we will explore the causes and symptoms of joint pain to gain a better understanding of this condition.

Causes of Joint Pain:

Joint pain can be a debilitating condition that can significantly impact an individual's quality of life. It can affect any joint in the body, including the knees, hips, shoulders, and elbows. Joint pain can be caused by a variety of factors, including injury, arthritis, infection, and autoimmune disorders. In this article, we will discuss the various causes of joint pain.

1. Arthritis: Arthritis is one of the most common causes of joint pain. There are many types of arthritis, but the most common types are osteoarthritis and rheumatoid arthritis. Osteoarthritis is a degenerative condition that affects the cartilage that cushions the joints. Rheumatoid arthritis is an autoimmune disorder that causes inflammation in the joints, leading to pain, stiffness, and swelling.

2. Injury: Injury is another common cause of joint pain. This can include sprains, strains, and fractures. Sports injuries, car accidents, and falls are some of the most common causes of joint injuries. Joint injuries can lead to inflammation and pain, and they can also cause long-term damage to the joints.

3. Infection: Infections can also cause joint pain. This can include bacterial, viral, and fungal infections. Joint infections can occur when bacteria or other pathogens enter the joint through the bloodstream or from an open wound. Symptoms of a joint infection may include pain, swelling, redness, and fever.

4. Gout: Gout is a type of arthritis that is caused by the buildup of uric acid crystals in the joints. Gout typically affects the big toe, but it can also affect other joints in the body. Symptoms of gout include sudden onset of intense pain, swelling, and redness in the affected joint.

5. Autoimmune Disorders: Autoimmune disorders such as lupus and psoriatic arthritis can also cause joint pain. These disorders occur when the immune system attacks the body's tissues, leading to inflammation and damage to the joints. Symptoms of autoimmune disorders can vary, but they may include joint pain, stiffness, and swelling.

6. Overuse: Overuse can also cause joint pain. This can include repetitive motions such as typing, playing an instrument, or participating in sports. Overuse can cause inflammation and pain in the joints, leading to conditions such as tennis elbow, golfer's elbow, and runner's knee.

7. Genetics: Genetics can also play a role in the development of joint pain. Certain genetic factors can make an individual more susceptible to conditions such as arthritis and other joint disorders. Individuals with a family history of joint pain may be at an increased risk of developing joint pain themselves.

8. Age: Age is another factor that can contribute to joint pain. As we age, the cartilage in our joints may start to wear down, leading to pain, stiffness, and limited mobility. Osteoarthritis is more common in older adults, and it can cause significant joint pain and discomfort.

9. Obesity: Obesity can also increase the risk of joint pain. Excess weight puts added stress on the joints, particularly the knees, hips, and ankles. Over time, this can cause wear and tear on the joints,

leading to pain and inflammation. Losing weight through diet and exercise can help to reduce joint pain and improve overall joint health.

10. Poor Posture: Poor posture can also contribute to joint pain, particularly in the neck, shoulders, and back. Sitting or standing in the same position for ext extended periods puts added stress on the joints, leading to pain and discomfort. Maintaining good posture and taking frequent breaks to stretch and move can help to reduce joint pain caused by poor posture.

11. Hormonal Changes: Hormonal changes can also play a role in joint pain. Women may experience joint pain during certain times of their menstrual cycle or menopause. This is due to changes in hormone levels that can affect joint inflammation and pain.

12. Medications: Certain medications can also cause joint pain as a side effect. This can include medications used to treat cancer, as well as drugs used to lower cholesterol or blood pressure. If you are experiencing joint pain while taking medication, it is important to speak with your healthcare provider.

13. Inactivity: Finally, inactivity can also contribute to joint pain. A sedentary lifestyle can cause the muscles and joints to become weak, leading to pain and stiffness. Regular exercise can help to strengthen the muscles and improve joint mobility, reducing the risk of joint pain.

In summary, joint pain can be caused by a wide range of factors, including injury, arthritis, infection, autoimmune disorders, overuse, genetics, age, obesity, poor posture, hormonal changes, medication,s and inactivity. If you are experiencing joint pain, it is important to speak with your healthcare provider to determine the underlying cause and develop an appropriate treatment plan. Early intervention can help to prevent long-term damage to the joints and improve your overall quality of life By understanding the underlying causes of joint pain, individuals can take steps to reduce their risk and improve their joint health. This may include maintaining a healthy weight, practicing good posture, exercising regularly, and seeking medical treatment when necessary.

Symptoms of Joint Pain:

Joint pain is a common health condition that affects millions of people worldwide. It is characterized by discomfort, aches, and soreness in any joint of the body, ranging from mild to severe. Joint pain can be caused by several factors such as injury, inflammation, infection, age-related wear and tear, and autoimmune diseases. The symptoms of joint pain can vary from person to person, depending on the underlying cause and the severity of the condition.

Here are some of the most common symptoms of joint pain:

1. Pain and discomfort: Joint pain is often accompanied by pain and discomfort, which can range from mild to severe. The pain can be dull, aching, stabbing, or burning, and can occur in one or more joints. The pain may also be constant or intermittent, depending on the underlying cause.

2. Swelling: Joint pain can cause swelling and inflammation in the affected joint. This can make the joint appear red, warm, and tender to the touch. Swelling can occur in any joint, but it is most commonly seen in the knee, ankle, and wrist.

3. Stiffness: Joint pain can cause stiffness and limited mobility in the affected joint. This can make it difficult to move the joint freely, and can also cause a feeling of stiffness or rigidity in the joint.

4. Weakness: Joint pain can cause weakness in the affected joint, making it difficult to perform daily activities such as walking, standing, or lifting objects.

5. Cracking and popping sounds: Joint pain can cause cracking and popping sounds in the affected joint. This is often due to the movement of the joint, which can cause the bones to rub against each other.

6. Fever: Joint pain accompanied by fever can indicate an underlying infection or inflammation in the joint. This can cause the joint to feel hot and tender to the touch.

7. Fatigue: Joint pain can cause fatigue and a general feeling of malaise. This can make it difficult to perform daily activities and can also affect a person's mood and overall quality of life.

8. Numbness and tingling: Joint pain can cause numbness and tingling in the affected joint or surrounding area. This can be a sign of nerve damage or compression, which requires immediate medical attention.

In conclusion, joint pain is a common condition that can affect anyone, regardless of age or gender. The symptoms of joint pain can vary, depending on the underlying cause and the severity of the condition. If you are experiencing joint pain, it is important to seek medical attention to determine the underlying cause and receive appropriate treatment.

Diagnosis of Joint Pain:

Proper diagnosis is crucial to determine the underlying cause of joint pain and develop an appropriate treatment plan.

Here are some of the steps involved in the diagnosis of joint pain:

1. Medical history: The first step in diagnosing joint pain is to take a detailed medical history. The doctor will ask questions about the location, duration, and severity of the pain. They will also ask

about any previous injuries, medical conditions, or surgeries. This information will help the doctor to narrow down the possible causes of joint pain.

2. Physical examination: The doctor will perform a physical examination of the affected joint to check for any visible signs of inflammation, swelling, or tenderness. They may also assess the range of motion of the joint and ask the patient to perform certain movements to evaluate joint function.

3. Imaging tests: Imaging tests such as X-rays, MRI, or CT scans can provide detailed images of the bones, joints, and surrounding tissues. These tests can help to identify any structural abnormalities, such as fractures, dislocations, or cartilage damage. They can also detect signs of arthritis or other degenerative diseases.

4. Blood tests: Blood tests can help to detect signs of inflammation or infection in the body. They can also measure the levels of certain antibodies or proteins that are associated with autoimmune diseases such as rheumatoid arthritis.

5. Joint fluid analysis: In some cases, the doctor may perform a joint fluid analysis to check for signs of infection, inflammation, or other abnormalities. This involves removing a small sample of fluid from the affected joint and examining it under a microscope.

6. Diagnostic injections: Diagnostic injections involve injecting a small amount of a local anesthetic or steroid medication into the affected joint to determine if the pain is coming from the joint itself or surrounding tissues. If the injection provides temporary relief, it can confirm the diagnosis of joint pain and help guide further treatment.

7. Evaluation of other symptoms: Joint pain can be accompanied by other symptoms such as fever, fatigue, or weight loss. The presence of these symptoms can provide clues as to the underlying cause of joint pain and help guide the diagnostic process.

8. Consultation with specialists: Depending on the suspected cause of joint pain, the doctor may refer the patient to a specialist such as a rheumatologist, orthopedist, or neurologist. These specialists have expertise in diagnosing and treating specific conditions that can cause joint pain.

9. Functional assessments: In some cases, functional assessments such as gait analysis or muscle strength testing may be performed to evaluate the impact of joint pain on mobility and function.

10. Patient input: Patients should be encouraged to provide detailed descriptions of their symptoms and any factors that may exacerbate or alleviate their joint pain. This information can help the doctor to make an accurate diagnosis and develop a personalized treatment plan.

It is important to note that the diagnosis of joint pain can be complex and may require multiple diagnostic tests and consultations with specialists. In some cases, the cause of joint pain may remain unclear despite extensive testing. However, with a thorough evaluation and individualized treatment plan, most patients can achieve significant relief from joint pain and improve their overall quality of life.

Chapter two:
Traditional Remedies for Joint Pain: A Historical Perspective

Traditional Remedies:

For centuries, people have sought relief from joint pain through various traditional remedies. These remedies passed down through generations, have been used to treat a wide range of joint conditions, from minor aches and pains to chronic diseases like arthritis. In this chapter, we will explore the historical roots of these traditional remedies and their role in modern-day joint pain management.

Ancient Times: Ayurveda and Traditional Chinese Medicine

The use of traditional remedies for joint pain dates back thousands of years. In ancient India, Ayurvedic medicine was developed, which uses natural herbs and plants to treat a wide range of ailments, including joint pain. According to Ayurveda, joint pain is caused by an imbalance in the body's three doshas: vata, pitta, and kapha. To restore balance, Ayurvedic practitioners use a combination of herbal remedies, massage, and dietary changes.

Similarly, in ancient China, Traditional Chinese Medicine (TCM) was developed, which uses a holistic approach to healing that focuses on restoring the body's balance. TCM practitioners use a variety of remedies, including herbal remedies, acupuncture, and massage, to treat joint pain. They believe that joint pain is caused by blockages in the body's energy pathways, known as meridians. By unblocking these meridians, they can restore balance to the body and relieve joint pain.

Middle Ages: European Herbal Remedies

During the Middle Ages in Europe, herbal remedies became popular for treating joint pain. Many of these remedies were based on the writings of the ancient Greek physician Hippocrates, who believed in the healing power of nature. Herbal remedies like willow bark and meadowsweet were used to relieve joint pain, as they contain salicin, a natural pain reliever. Other herbs like ginger and turmeric were also used for their anti-inflammatory properties.

Renaissance: European Medical Advances

In the Renaissance period, European medical advances led to the development of new treatments for joint pain. The Swiss physician Paracelsus, for example, believed that many illnesses were caused by mineral imbalances in the body. He developed a treatment for joint pain using mercury, which he believed could restore the body's balance.

At the same time, the Italian physician Andrea Cesalpino developed a treatment for joint pain using opium, which he believed could relieve pain and inflammation. These treatments, while effective in some cases, were also dangerous and often led to serious side effects.

Modern Era: Integrative Medicine

In the modern era, traditional remedies for joint pain have continued to be used alongside modern medicine. This approach, known as integrative medicine, combines the best of both worlds, using traditional remedies alongside modern treatments like pain medication and physical therapy.

Many traditional remedies, like acupuncture and herbal remedies, have been scientifically proven to be effective in relieving joint pain. For example, a study published in the Journal of Clinical Rheumatology found that acupuncture was an effective treatment for knee osteoarthritis. Similarly, a study published in the journal Arthritis & Rheumatism found that ginger was effective in reducing joint pain in people with osteoarthritis.

Acupuncture is a form of traditional Chinese medicine that involves the insertion of thin needles into specific points of the body. Acupuncture is believed to stimulate the body's natural healing process and promote the flow of energy throughout the body. Many people have reported significant relief from joint pain after undergoing acupuncture treatment.

Natural Remedies:

Natural remedies for joint pain have become increasingly popular in recent years, as more people seek safer and more effective alternatives to conventional medicine. These natural remedies often involve the use of herbs, essential oils, supplements, and lifestyle changes to manage joint pain.

Herbs are a common natural remedy for joint pain. Many herbs contain anti-inflammatory and analgesic properties that can help reduce pain and inflammation in the joints. Some of the most commonly used herbs for joint pain include ginger, turmeric, willow bark, and boswellia. These herbs can be consumed in tea or supplement form or used topically in creams and salves.

Essential oils are another natural remedy for joint pain. Essential oils are highly concentrated plant extracts that contain powerful medicinal properties. Many essential oils have anti-inflammatory and pain-relieving properties that can help reduce joint pain. Some of the most commonly used essential oils for joint pain include peppermint, eucalyptus, lavender, and frankincense. These oils can be used topically or inhaled using a diffuser.

Yoga is another natural remedy for joint pain. Yoga involves a series of poses and movements that can help improve flexibility, strength, and balance. Yoga can be particularly helpful for people with joint pain because it is low-impact and gentle on the joints. Some yoga poses are specifically designed to help reduce joint pain, such as the downward dog and the pigeon pose.

Diet and nutrition can also play a significant role in joint health. A diet rich in anti-inflammatory foods, such as fruits, vegetables, and fatty fish, can help reduce inflammation in the joints and improve overall joint health. Supplements like glucosamine and chondroitin can also be helpful for people with joint pain.

Lifestyle changes can also be beneficial for managing joint pain. Exercise, for example, can help improve joint mobility and reduce pain. Low-impact exercises like swimming and cycling are particularly helpful for people with joint pain. Getting enough sleep and reducing stress can also help improve joint health.

Traditional remedies for joint pain have a long and rich history, dating back thousands of years. While some of these remedies may seem outdated, many are still used today alongside modern treatments. Integrative medicine, which combines traditional and modern approaches to healing, is becoming increasingly popular, as people seek a more holistic approach to managing their joint pain.

research is needed to fully understand the mechanisms behind these traditional remedies and to determine their efficacy in treating different types of joint pain. However, the use of traditional remedies has been shown to have few side effects, making them a safe and natural alternative to conventional medication.

It's important to note that not all traditional remedies are safe, and some can interact with other medications or have adverse effects. It's important to consult with a healthcare provider before using any traditional remedies for joint pain, especially if you are taking other medications or have underlying health conditions.

In addition to the use of traditional remedies, lifestyle changes can also play a significant role in managing joint pain. Maintaining a healthy weight, exercising regularly, and eating a nutritious diet can all help to reduce inflammation and improve joint health. Other complementary therapies, such as massage and physical therapy, can also be effective in relieving joint pain.

In conclusion, traditional remedies for joint pain have been used for centuries and continue to be used today alongside modern medicine. While more research is needed to fully understand their efficacy, they offer a safe and natural alternative to conventional medication. Integrative medicine, which combines traditional and modern approaches to healing, offers a holistic approach to managing joint pain that can help improve overall health and well-being. Natural remedies for joint pain,n on the other hand, include herbs, essential oils, acupuncture, yoga, diet, nutrition, and lifestyle changes and can be highly effective in managing joint pain. By incorporating these natural remedies into your daily routine, you can reduce joint pain and improve your overall joint health.

Chapter three:
The Role of Inflammation in Joint Pain and How to Combat It Naturally

Joint pain is a common ailment that affects millions of people worldwide. It can range from mild discomfort to severe pain that limits mobility and reduces quality of life. One of the major causes of joint pain is inflammation, a natural response of the body to injury or infection. While inflammation is necessary for healing, chronic inflammation can lead to tissue damage and contribute to the development of chronic conditions such as osteoarthritis, rheumatoid arthritis, and gout.

In this chapter, we will explore the role of inflammation in joint pain and how to combat it naturally.

Understanding Inflammation

Inflammation is the body's natural response to injury, infection, or foreign substances. When the body detects a threat, such as a virus, bacteria, or physical injury, it triggers an immune response that includes the release of cytokines and other immune cells. These cytokines help to recruit immune cells to the site of injury or infection to fight off the invaders and repair damaged tissue.

While acute inflammation is a necessary part of the healing process, chronic inflammation can be harmful. Chronic inflammation occurs when the immune system stays activated for extended periods, causing damage to healthy tissue. Chronic inflammation can lead to tissue destruction, scarring, and the development of chronic diseases such as heart disease, cancer, and autoimmune disorders.

Inflammation and Joint Pain

Joint pain is often caused by inflammation in the joints. When the immune system mistakenly attacks healthy tissue in the joints, it can cause inflammation and damage to the joint cartilage, leading to joint pain and stiffness. Inflammatory joint conditions, such as rheumatoid arthritis, psoriatic arthritis, and gout, are examples of chronic inflammatory conditions that can cause joint pain.

Inflammation can also contribute to the development of osteoarthritis, the most common form of arthritis. Osteoarthritis is a degenerative joint disease that occurs when the protective cartilage that cushions the joints breaks down over time. When the cartilage breaks down, the bones in the joint can rub against each other, causing pain, stiffness, and inflammation.

How to Combat Inflammation Naturally

While medication can be an effective way to reduce inflammation and joint pain, there are also natural ways to combat inflammation. Lifestyle changes, such as diet and exercise, can help to reduce chronic inflammation and improve joint health.

Diet

A healthy diet can help to reduce inflammation in the body. Foods that are high in antioxidants, such as fruits, vegetables, nuts, and seeds, can help to reduce inflammation by neutralizing free radicals, which can cause damage to cells and contribute to inflammation.

Omega-3 fatty acids, found in fatty fish such as salmon, mackerel, and sardines, have anti-inflammatory properties and can help to reduce joint pain and stiffness. Other anti-inflammatory foods include turmeric, ginger, garlic, and green tea.

On the other hand, processed foods, sugary drinks, and foods high in saturated and trans fats can contribute to inflammation and worsen joint pain. Reducing the consumption of these foods can help to improve joint health.

Exercise

Regular exercise can also help to reduce inflammation and joint pain. Exercise helps to strengthen the muscles and improve joint mobility, reducing the stress on the joints. It also helps to reduce weight, which can relieve pressure on the joints and reduce inflammation.

Low-impact exercises, such as walking, swimming, and cycling, are ideal for people with joint pain as they are less likely to cause further damage to the joints. Strength training exercises can also help to improve joint health by strengthening the muscles around the joints.

Other Natural Remedies

In addition to diet and exercise, other natural remedies can help to reduce inflammation and joint pain. These include:

1. Heat and Cold Therapy: Applying heat or cold to the affected area can help to reduce inflammation and alleviate joint pain. Heat therapy, such as a warm towel or heating pad, can help to increase blood flow and relax the muscles. Cold therapy, such as an ice pack or cold compress, can help to reduce swelling and numb the pain.

2. Massage: Massage therapy can help to improve joint mobility and reduce inflammation by increasing blood flow and relaxing the muscles. It can also help to reduce stress and promote relaxation.

3. Acupuncture: Acupuncture is a traditional Chinese medicine technique that involves inserting thin needles into specific points on the body. It is effective in reducing inflammation and alleviating joint pain.

4. Supplements: Certain supplements can help to reduce inflammation and improve joint health. Glucosamine and chondroitin are commonly used supplements for joint health, as

they help to rebuild and protect joint cartilage. Omega-3 fatty acids and turmeric supplements are also effective in reducing inflammation.

5. Mind-Body Techniques: Mind-body techniques, such as yoga, meditation, and tai chi, can help to reduce inflammation and improve joint health by reducing stress and promoting relaxation.

Conclusion

Inflammation plays a significant role in joint pain and can lead to the development of chronic conditions such as arthritis. While medication can be effective in reducing inflammation and joint pain, natural remedies such as diet and exercise can also help to improve joint health and reduce inflammation. By incorporating these natural remedies into your daily routine, you can reduce inflammation and improve joint health, leading to a better quality of life.

Chapter four:
The Science of Herbal Medicine: Effective Plants for Joint Pain Relief

Herbal medicine has been used for centuries to treat various ailments, including joint pain. Many plants have been found to contain compounds that have anti-inflammatory, analgesic, and antioxidant properties, which can help reduce joint pain and inflammation. In this chapter, we will explore some of the most effective plants for joint pain relief and the scientific evidence supporting their use.

Turmeric

Turmeric is a spice commonly used in Indian cuisine and has been used in Ayurvedic medicine for centuries to treat various ailments, including joint pain. The active compound in turmeric is curcumin, which has potent anti-inflammatory and antioxidant properties. Studies have shown that curcumin can reduce joint pain and stiffness in people with osteoarthritis and rheumatoid arthritis.

In a randomized, double-blind, placebo-controlled study, 45 people with osteoarthritis of the knee were given either 1,500 mg of turmeric extract or a placebo for four weeks. The group that received the turmeric extract experienced a significant reduction in joint pain and stiffness compared to the placebo group.

Ginger

Ginger is another spice commonly used in cooking and has been used in traditional medicine for centuries to treat various ailments, including joint pain. The active compounds in ginger, gingerols, and schools, have potent anti-inflammatory and analgesic properties. Studies have shown that ginger can reduce joint pain and inflammation in people with osteoarthritis and rheumatoid arthritis.

In a randomized, double-blind, placebo-controlled study, 247 people with osteoarthritis of the knee were given either a placebo or 255 mg of ginger extract twice daily for six weeks. The group that received the ginger extract experienced a significant reduction in knee pain compared to the placebo group.

Boswellia

Boswellia, also known as Indian frankincense, is a tree native to India and has been used in Ayurvedic medicine for centuries to treat various ailments, including joint pain. The active compounds in boswellia, boswellic acids, have potent anti-inflammatory properties. Studies have shown that boswellia can reduce joint pain and inflammation in people with osteoarthritis and rheumatoid arthritis.

In a randomized, double-blind, placebo-controlled study, 75 people with osteoarthritis of the knee were given either a placebo or 100 mg of boswellia extract three times daily for eight weeks. The group that received the Boswellia extract experienced a significant reduction in knee pain and stiffness compared to the placebo group.

Devil's Claw

Devil's Claw is a plant native to southern Africa and has been used in traditional medicine for centuries to treat various ailments, including joint pain. The active compounds in devil's claw, harpagosides, have potent anti-inflammatory and analgesic properties. Studies have shown that devil's claw can reduce joint pain and inflammation in people with osteoarthritis and rheumatoid arthritis.

In a randomized, double-blind, placebo-controlled study, 89 people with osteoarthritis of the hip or knee were given either a placebo or 2,610 mg of devil's claw extract daily for six weeks. The group that received the devil's claw extract experienced a significant reduction in hip and knee pain compared to the placebo group.

Willow Bark

Willow bark is a plant native to Europe and Asia and has been used in traditional medicine for centuries to treat various ailments, including joint pain. The active compound in willow bark, salicin, is a natural anti-inflammatory and analgesic. Studies have shown that willow bark can reduce joint pain and inflammation in people with osteoarthritis and rheumatoid arthritis.

In a randomized, double-blind, placebo-controlled study, 127 people with osteoarthritis of the hip or knee were given either a placebo or 240 mg of willow bark extract twice daily for six weeks. The group that received the willow bark extract experienced a significant reduction in joint pain and stiffness compared to the placebo group.

Green Tea

Green tea is a beverage made from the leaves of the Camellia sinensis plant and has been consumed for centuries in traditional medicine for various health benefits, including joint pain relief. The active compound in green tea, epigallocatechin-3-gallate (EGCG), has potent anti-inflammatory and antioxidant properties. Studies have shown that green tea can reduce joint pain and inflammation in people with osteoarthritis and rheumatoid arthritis.

In a randomized, double-blind, placebo-controlled study, 60 people with rheumatoid arthritis were given either a placebo or 500 mg of green tea extract daily for 12 weeks. The group that received the green tea extract experienced a significant reduction in joint pain and stiffness compared to the placebo group.

Conclusion

Herbal medicine offers a promising alternative or complementary treatment for joint pain relief. The plants discussed in this chapter are effective in reducing joint pain and inflammation in various clinical studies. However, it is important to note that herbal medicine should not replace conventional medical treatment, and it is important to consult a healthcare professional before using any herbal remedies. Additionally, the dosage, quality, and safety of herbal remedies should be carefully considered, as some plants may have side effects or interact with medications. Overall, herbal medicine can be a valuable tool in the management of joint pain, and further research is needed to explore the full potential of these natural remedies.

Chapter five:
Aromatherapy for Joint Pain: Essential Oils and Their Benefits

Joint pain can be a debilitating condition that affects people of all ages. It can be caused by a variety of factors such as injury, arthritis, or simply aging. While there are several treatment options available, many people turn to alternative therapies such as aromatherapy for relief. Essential oils, which are extracted from various plants, have been used for centuries for their therapeutic properties. In this chapter, we will discuss the benefits of essential oils for joint pain and how to use them.

What are Essential Oils?

Essential oils are concentrated plant extracts that are derived from the leaves, flowers, stems, and roots of plants. They are often used in aromatherapy, which is a holistic healing approach that uses essential oils to promote physical and psychological well-being. Essential oils are known for their therapeutic properties such as anti-inflammatory, analgesic, and antispasmodic effects.

How Essential Oils Work

Essential oils contain volatile organic compounds (VOCs) that can penetrate the skin and enter the bloodstream. Once in the bloodstream, these compounds can have a variety of effects on the body. For example, some essential oils can help to reduce inflammation, while others can help to alleviate pain. Essential oils can also affect the nervous system and help to promote relaxation and reduce stress.

Benefits of Essential Oils for Joint Pain

Essential oils can be used to help relieve joint pain in a variety of ways. Here are some of the most common benefits of essential oils for joint pain:

1. Anti-inflammatory Properties: Several essential oils, such as peppermint, eucalyptus, and frankincense, have anti-inflammatory properties. These oils can help to reduce inflammation and swelling in the joints, which can help to relieve pain.

2. Analgesic Properties: Many essential oils, including lavender, ginger, and clove, have analgesic properties. These oils can help to reduce pain by blocking pain signals in the nervous system.

3. Muscle Relaxant Properties: Essential oils such as chamomile and lavender have muscle-relaxant properties. These oils can help to relax tight muscles and reduce muscle spasms, which can be beneficial for people with joint pain.

4. Stress Reduction: Stress can exacerbate joint pain, so reducing stress levels can help manage joint pain. Essential oils such as lavender, bergamot, and ylang-ylang have been shown to have stress-reducing effects.

5. Improved Sleep: Essential oils such as lavender and chamomile can also help to improve sleep quality. Getting enough restful sleep is important for people with joint pain as it can help to reduce pain levels and improve overall well-being.

How to Use Essential Oils for Joint Pain

There are several ways to use essential oils for joint pain. Here are some of the most common methods:

1. Topical Application: Essential oils can be applied topically to the affected joint. Dilute the essential oil with a carrier oil such as coconut or jojoba oil, and then massage it into the skin over the affected joint.

2. Aromatherapy Diffuser: Aromatherapy diffusers are a popular way to use essential oils. Add a few drops of essential oil to a diffuser, and let it run for several hours in the room where you spend the most time.

3. Bath: Add a few drops of essential oil to a warm bath and soak for at least 20 minutes. This can be a relaxing and effective way to use essential oils for joint pain.

4. Compress: Add a few drops of essential oil to a bowl of warm water, soak a cloth in the water, and then apply the cloth to the affected joint.

5. Massage: A gentle massage with essential oils can also help to alleviate joint pain. Dilute the essential oil with a carrier oil and then massage it into the affected joint.

6. Topical Patches: Essential oil patches can be placed directly on the affected joint for long-lasting relief. These patches typically contain a blend of essential oils that have anti-inflammatory and analgesic properties.

7. Roll-Ons: Essential oil roll-ons are convenient and easy to use. Simply apply the roll-on to the affected joint as needed throughout the day.

Best Essential Oils for Joint Pain

Many essential oils can be helpful for joint pain, but some are more effective than others. Here are some of the best essential oils for joint pain:

Peppermint: Peppermint oil has anti-inflammatory and analgesic properties. It can help to reduce inflammation and relieve pain in the joints.

Eucalyptus: Eucalyptus oil has anti-inflammatory properties and can help to reduce swelling in the joints.

Frankincense: Frankincense oil has anti-inflammatory properties and can help to reduce joint pain and stiffness.

Lavender: Lavender oil has analgesic and muscle relaxant properties. It can help to reduce pain and muscle tension in the joints.

Ginger: Ginger oil has analgesic properties and can help to reduce pain and inflammation in the joints.

Chamomile: Chamomile oil has muscle relaxant properties and can help to reduce muscle spasms and tension in the joints.

Clove: Clove oil has analgesic properties and can help to reduce pain and inflammation in the joints.

Rosemary: Rosemary oil has analgesic and anti-inflammatory properties. It can help to reduce pain and inflammation in the joints.

Safety Precautions

While essential oils can be a safe and effective treatment for joint pain, it is important to use them correctly and safely. Here are some safety precautions to keep in mind when using essential oils:

1. Dilute essential oils with carrier oil before applying them to the skin. Essential oils can be irritating to the skin and can cause allergic reactions.

2. Do not ingest essential oils. Some essential oils can be toxic if ingested, and ingesting essential oils can cause serious health problems.

3. Keep essential oils out of reach of children and pets.

4. Use essential oils in a well-ventilated area to avoid inhaling too much of the oil.

5. Talk to your doctor before using essential oils if you are pregnant, nursing, or have a medical condition.

Conclusion

Essential oils can be a safe and effective treatment for joint pain. They have a variety of therapeutic properties that can help to reduce inflammation, alleviate pain, and promote relaxation. When using essential oils for joint pain, it is important to choose the right oils and use them correctly and safely. By incorporating essential oils into your treatment plan, you may be able to find relief from joint pain and improve your overall well-being.

Chapter six:
Holistic Approaches to Joint Pain Management: Acupuncture,
Massage, and More

Joint pain is a common problem that can greatly impact an individual's quality of life. While traditional treatments such as painkillers and physical therapy can be effective, many people seek out alternative therapies for relief. Holistic approaches, such as acupuncture and massage, have been gaining popularity in recent years. These therapies address not only the physical symptoms but also the emotional and mental aspects of pain. This chapter will explore some of the most effective holistic approaches to joint pain management.

Acupuncture

Acupuncture is an ancient Chinese healing practice that involves inserting thin needles into specific points on the body. The practice is based on the concept of qi (pronounced "chee"), which is the flow of energy through the body. According to traditional Chinese medicine, joint pain is caused by a blockage or imbalance of it. Acupuncture aims to restore balance and improve the flow of it.

There is a growing body of research supporting the use of acupuncture for joint pain. A meta-analysis of 29 randomized controlled trials found that acupuncture was effective in reducing pain and improving function in patients with osteoarthritis of the knee. Another study found that acupuncture was as effective as painkillers in relieving pain in patients with knee osteoarthritis.

Acupuncture is generally considered safe when performed by a qualified practitioner. However, it is important to note that it may not be suitable for everyone. Individuals with bleeding disorders or those taking blood thinners should avoid acupuncture, as there is a risk of bleeding or bruising at the insertion site. It is also important to seek out a licensed acupuncturist and to discuss any concerns with your healthcare provider.

Massage

Massage is a therapeutic practice that involves manipulating the soft tissues of the body, including muscles, tendons, and ligaments. It is often used to relieve muscle tension and promote relaxation, but it can also be effective in reducing joint pain.

There are several different types of massage, each with its techniques and benefits. A Swedish massage is a gentle form of massage that involves long strokes, kneading, and circular movements. Deep tissue massage, on the other hand, uses more pressure and targets deeper layers of muscle tissue.

Research has shown that massage can be effective in reducing joint pain. A systematic review of 12 randomized controlled trials found that massage was effective in reducing pain and improving function in patients with osteoarthritis (3). Another study found that massage was as effective as physical therapy in reducing pain and improving function in patients with knee osteoarthritis (4).

Like acupuncture, massage is generally considered safe when performed by a qualified practitioner. However, it may not be suitable for everyone. Individuals with certain conditions, such as osteoporosis or rheumatoid arthritis, may require special precautions or modifications to the massage technique.

Yoga

Yoga is a mind-body practice that combines physical postures, breathing techniques, and meditation. It is effective in reducing stress, improving flexibility, and promoting relaxation. It can also be effective in reducing joint pain.

Several studies have shown that yoga can be effective in reducing joint pain. A randomized controlled trial of 75 patients with knee osteoarthritis found that a 12-week yoga program was effective in reducing pain and improving function (5). Another study found that a 6-week yoga program was effective in reducing pain and improving quality of life in patients with rheumatoid arthritis (6).

It is important to note that not all yoga poses are suitable for individuals with joint pain. It is important to seek out a qualified yoga instructor who can help modify poses to suit your individual needs.

Mind-Body Techniques

Mind-body techniques, such as meditation and biofeedback, can be effective in reducing joint pain by reducing stress and promoting relaxation. Chronic pain can often lead to increased stress and anxiety, which can in turn exacerbate the pain. Mind-body techniques can help break this cycle by promoting relaxation and reducing stress levels.

Meditation is a practice that involves focusing the mind on a particular object or activity, such as the breath or a mantra. It is effective in reducing stress and anxiety, and may also help reduce joint pain. A study of 43 patients with rheumatoid arthritis found that a 10-week mindfulness meditation program was effective in reducing pain and improving quality of life (7).

Biofeedback is a technique that involves using electronic devices to monitor and provide feedback on physiological processes, such as heart rate and muscle tension. It can be used to help individuals learn to control their physiological responses and promote relaxation. A study of 18 patients with knee osteoarthritis found that biofeedback was effective in reducing pain and improving function (8).

Other Holistic Approaches

Many other holistic approaches can be effective in reducing joint pain. These include:

Dietary changes: Certain foods, such as those high in omega-3 fatty acids and antioxidants, may help reduce inflammation and joint pain.

Herbal remedies: Some herbs, such as turmeric and ginger, have anti-inflammatory properties and may help reduce joint pain.

Chiropractic care: Chiropractors use manual manipulation to help restore joint function and reduce pain.

Acupressure: Acupressure involves applying pressure to specific points on the body to help restore balance and reduce pain.

It is important to note that while these approaches can be effective, they should not be used as a substitute for medical treatment. It is important to consult with a healthcare provider before starting any new treatment or therapy.

Overall, a holistic approach to joint pain management involves taking a comprehensive view of the individual and addressing all aspects of their health and well-being. This can include physical, emotional, and mental factors, as well as lifestyle choices such as diet and exercise.

It is important to note that while holistic approaches can be effective in reducing joint pain, they may not be appropriate for everyone. It is important to consult with a healthcare provider to determine the best course of treatment based on an individual's specific needs and medical history.

In addition, it is important to recognize that holistic approaches should not be used as a substitute for medical treatment. While these approaches can be effective in reducing joint pain and improving overall health, they should be used in conjunction with traditional medical treatments as needed.

In conclusion, a holistic approach to joint pain management can be a valuable tool for those looking to improve their overall health and reduce joint pain. By addressing all aspects of an individual's health and well-being, holistic approaches can provide a more comprehensive and sustainable solution to joint pain than traditional treatments alone. With the guidance of a qualified practitioner and in consultation with a healthcare provider, individuals can explore the many holistic approaches available and find the best options for their specific needs

Chapter seven:
Yoga and Tai Chi for Joint Health and Pain Relief

Yoga and Tai Chi are two ancient practices that have been used for centuries to promote physical and mental well-being. They are both low-impact, gentle forms of exercise that can help to relieve joint pain, reduce stress and anxiety, and improve overall joint health. In this chapter, we will explore the benefits of these two practices for joint health and pain relief, as well as provide tips for getting started with yoga and Tai Chi.

The Benefits of Yoga for Joint Health

Yoga is a form of exercise that involves stretching, strengthening, and balancing the body through a series of poses or asanas. Many of these poses can be adapted to accommodate different levels of flexibility and joint health, making it an ideal form of exercise for people with joint pain or arthritis.

One of the primary benefits of yoga for joint health is improved flexibility. Many of the poses in yoga focus on stretching the muscles and connective tissues around the joints, which can help to increase the range of motion and reduce stiffness. Regular practice of yoga can also help to improve balance and coordination, which can be especially helpful for people with joint pain who may be at risk of falling.

Yoga also has a calming effect on the body and mind, which can help to reduce stress and anxiety. Stress and anxiety can contribute to joint pain by increasing inflammation in the body and worsening symptoms of arthritis. By reducing stress levels, yoga can help to reduce inflammation and improve overall joint health.

The Benefits of Tai Chi for Joint Health

Tai Chi is a gentle form of exercise that involves slow, flowing movements that are designed to improve balance, coordination, and flexibility. It is often described as a moving meditation and has been used for centuries to promote physical and mental well-being.

Like yoga, Tai Chi is low-impact and gentle on the joints, making it an ideal form of exercise for people with joint pain or arthritis. The slow, flowing movements of Tai Chi help to increase flexibility and range of motion, while also improving balance and coordination.

Tai Chi has also been shown to have several mental health benefits, including reducing stress and anxiety, improving mood, and promoting relaxation. By reducing stress levels, Tai Chi can help to reduce inflammation and improve overall joint health.

Getting Started with Yoga and Tai Chi

If you are interested in trying yoga or Tai Chi to improve your joint health, there are a few things to keep in mind.

First, it is important to talk to your doctor before starting any new exercise program, especially if you have joint pain or arthritis. Your doctor can help you determine if yoga or Tai Chi is safe for you, and may be able to recommend specific poses or modifications to accommodate your needs.

Once you have the green light from your doctor, it is important to find a qualified instructor who can help you learn the proper form and technique for each pose. Look for an instructor who has experience working with people with joint pain or arthritis, and who can provide modifications or alternative poses as needed.

When starting with yoga or Tai Chi, it is important to take it slow and listen to your body. Do not push yourself too hard, and if a pose feels uncomfortable or painful, back off or ask your instructor for help.

specifically, yoga and Tai Chi can help to improve joint health by increasing flexibility, strengthening the muscles around the joints, improving balance and coordination, reducing inflammation, and promoting relaxation and stress reduction.

When it comes to practicing yoga for joint health, there are a variety of poses that can be particularly helpful. For example, poses such as the Warrior series and Downward Facing Dog can help to stretch and strengthen the muscles in the legs, hips, and back, which can help to reduce joint pain and stiffness. Other poses, such as the Cat-Cow stretch and the Child's Pose, can help to improve flexibility and reduce tension in the neck and spine.

Similarly, Tai Chi involves a series of gentle, flowing movements that can be particularly effective for improving joint health. Some of the most common movements in Tai Chi include the "Grasp Sparrow's Tail" and "Brush Knee and Twist Step," both of which involve gentle, flowing movements that help to improve balance, coordination, and flexibility.

Ultimately, the key to getting the most benefit from yoga and Tai Chi for joint health is to find a practice that works for you and stick with it. Whether you prefer to practice on your own at home or in a group class setting, consistency is key. By incorporating yoga or Tai Chi into your daily routine, you can improve joint health, reduce joint pain, and enjoy all the benefits that these ancient practices have to offer.

Finally, it is important to be consistent with your practice. Both yoga and Tai Chi are most effective when practiced regularly, so aim to practice at least a few times a week to see the most benefit.

Conclusion

Yoga and Tai Chi are two gentle, low-impact forms of exercise that can be effective in improving joint health and reducing joint pain. Both practices focus on stretching, strengthening, and balancing the body, and can be adapted to accommodate different levels of flexibility and joint health. If you are interested in trying yoga or Tai Chi to improve your joint

**Chapter eight:
The Power of Mind-Body Medicine: Meditation and Relaxation
Techniques**

The mind and body are intimately connected, and this connection plays a critical role in our health and well-being. Mind-body medicine refers to practices that focus on the relationship between our thoughts, emotions, and physical health. Meditation and relaxation techniques are two such practices that have been shown to have a profound impact on our minds and body.

In this chapter, we will explore the power of mind-body medicine, specifically the benefits of meditation and relaxation techniques. We will examine the scientific evidence that supports the use of these practices and provide practical tips for incorporating them into your daily routine.

What is Mind-Body Medicine?

Mind-body medicine is a holistic approach to healthcare that recognizes the connection between the mind and body. It focuses on how our thoughts, emotions, and behaviors impact our physical health. Mind-body medicine encompasses a wide range of practices, including meditation, relaxation techniques, yoga, tai chi, and biofeedback.

These practices aim to reduce stress and promote relaxation, which in turn can help to reduce symptoms of many physical and mental health conditions. Mind-body medicine is often used in conjunction with traditional medical treatments, and it can be an effective complement to these treatments.

The Benefits of Meditation

Meditation is a technique that involves training the mind to focus and quieting the constant chatter that goes on in our heads. It has been

practiced for thousands of years in various cultures and religions and has
been shown to have numerous benefits for both the mind and body.

Reduced Stress and Anxiety

Meditation has been shown to reduce levels of the stress hormone cortisol.
This can help to reduce feelings of stress and anxiety, which can have a
positive impact on both mental and physical health. Studies have also
shown that meditation can help to reduce symptoms of anxiety disorders,
such as generalized anxiety disorder and social anxiety disorder.

Improved Emotional Well-being

Meditation has been shown to increase positive emotions, such as
happiness and contentment, and reduce negative emotions, such as anger
and sadness. It can also improve overall emotional well-being, helping
people to feel more in control of their thoughts and emotions.

Improved Concentration and Focus

Meditation can help to improve concentration and focus by training the
mind to stay present and focused on the task at hand. This can be
particularly beneficial for people with attention deficit hyperactivity disorder
(ADHD) or other conditions that impact focus and attention.

Reduced Symptoms of Depression

Studies have shown that meditation can help to reduce symptoms of
depression. It may be particularly beneficial when used in combination with
traditional treatments, such as medication and therapy.

Reduced Physical Symptoms of Stress

Meditation has been shown to reduce physical symptoms of stress, such as high blood pressure and tension headaches. It can also help to improve sleep, which can be disrupted by stress.

The Benefits of Relaxation Techniques

Relaxation techniques are practices that help to promote relaxation and reduce stress. There are many different types of relaxation techniques, including deep breathing, progressive muscle relaxation, and visualization.

Reduced Anxiety and Stress

Relaxation techniques can help to reduce feelings of anxiety and stress by promoting relaxation and reducing tension in the body. Studies have shown that these techniques can be particularly effective for people with generalized anxiety disorder and panic disorder.

Improved Sleep

Relaxation techniques can also help to improve sleep, which can be disrupted by stress and anxiety. Progressive muscle relaxation, in particular, is effective in promoting relaxation and improving sleep.

Reduced Pain

Relaxation techniques can help to reduce pain by promoting relaxation and reducing tension in the body. They may be particularly beneficial for people with chronic pain conditions, such as fibromyalgia and arthritis.

Improved Digestion

Relaxation techniques can also help to improve digestion by reducing tension in the muscles of the digestive tract. This can be particularly helpful for people with digestive disorders, such as irritable bowel syndrome (IBS).

Lowered Blood Pressure

Relaxation techniques, such as deep breathing and progressive muscle relaxation, have been shown to lower blood pressure. This can be beneficial for people with high blood pressure, which can increase the risk of heart disease and stroke.

Improved Immune Function

Stress can weaken the immune system, making it more difficult for the body to fight off illness and infection. Relaxation techniques have been shown to boost the immune system by reducing stress and promoting relaxation.

Practical Tips for Incorporating Mind-Body Medicine into Your Daily Routine

Incorporating mind-body medicine into your daily routine can be a powerful way to promote overall health and well-being. Here are some practical tips for incorporating meditation and relaxation techniques into your daily routine:

Start Small
If you're new to meditation or relaxation techniques, start small. Begin with just a few minutes each day and gradually increase the amount of time you spend practicing.

Find a Quiet Place
Find a quiet place where you can practice without distraction. This could be a dedicated meditation space or simply a quiet room in your home.

Use Guided Meditations
Guided meditations can be a helpful way to get started with meditation. There are many guided meditation apps and videos available online.

Practice Regularly

Regular practice is key to reaping the benefits of mind-body medicine. Set aside time each day to practice, even if it's just a few minutes.

Experiment with Different Techniques

There are many different types of meditation and relaxation techniques. Experiment with different techniques to find what works best for you.

Seek Professional Help if Needed

If you're struggling with a mental or physical health condition, seek professional help. Mind-body medicine can be a helpful complement to traditional treatments, but it should not be used as a substitute for medical care.

Conclusion

Meditation and relaxation techniques are powerful tools for promoting overall health and well-being. They can help to reduce stress and anxiety, improve emotional well-being, and reduce physical symptoms of stress. By incorporating these practices into your daily routine, you can harness the power of mind-body medicine and achieve greater balance and harmony in your life.

Chapter nine:
Diet and Nutrition for Joint Health: Foods to Eat and Avoid

Joint pain is a common ailment that affects millions of people worldwide. The health of our joints is essential for our mobility and overall quality of life. While many factors contribute to joint health, diet, and nutrition play a significant role in keeping our joints healthy and pain-free. In this chapter, we will discuss the foods to eat and avoid for joint health.

Foods to Eat for Joint Health

Fatty Fish: Fatty fish such as salmon, mackerel, and sardines are rich in omega-3 fatty acids. Omega-3 fatty acids have been shown to reduce inflammation in the body, which can help ease joint pain.

Nuts and Seeds: Nuts and seeds such as almonds, walnuts, and chia seeds are rich in omega-3 fatty acids, fiber, and antioxidants. These nutrients have anti-inflammatory properties and can help reduce joint pain.

Fruits and Vegetables: Fruits and vegetables are rich in antioxidants, vitamins, and minerals, which are essential for joint health. Dark leafy greens such as spinach and kale are rich in calcium, which is essential for strong bones.

Whole Grains: Whole grains such as brown rice, quinoa, and whole-wheat bread are rich in fiber, vitamins, and minerals. These nutrients are essential for overall health, including joint health.

Lean Proteins: Lean proteins such as chicken, turkey, and tofu are rich in amino acids, which are the building blocks of muscles and joints. Consuming lean proteins can help maintain healthy muscles and joints.

Foods to Avoid for Joint Health

Processed Foods: Processed foods such as chips, cookies, and candy are high in sugar and unhealthy fats. These foods can contribute to inflammation in the body, which can worsen joint pain.

Red Meat: Red meat is high in saturated fats, which can contribute to inflammation in the body. Consuming too much red meat can increase the risk of developing joint pain and other chronic diseases.

Fried Foods: Fried foods such as french fries and fried chicken are high in unhealthy fats, which can contribute to inflammation in the body. Consuming too many fried foods can worsen joint pain.

Sugary Beverages: Sugary beverages such as soda and energy drinks are high in sugar and can contribute to inflammation in the body. Consuming too many sugary beverages can increase the risk of developing joint pain and other chronic diseases.

Alcohol: Consuming too much alcohol can contribute to inflammation in the body, which can worsen joint pain. Alcohol can also interfere with the absorption of essential nutrients, which are essential for joint health.

In addition to the specific foods to eat and avoid, some general dietary guidelines can promote joint health. Here are some tips:

Stay hydrated: Drinking plenty of water can help keep joints lubricated and reduce the risk of injury.

Maintain a healthy weight: Excess weight puts pressure on joints, which can lead to pain and inflammation. Eating a healthy diet and exercising regularly can help maintain a healthy weight.

Limit salt intake: Consuming too much salt can lead to fluid retention and swelling, which can exacerbate joint pain.

Eat a variety of foods: Consuming a variety of foods ensures that you get all the nutrients your body needs for optimal joint health.

Consider supplements: Certain supplements, such as glucosamine and chondroitin, may help reduce joint pain and inflammation. However, it's important to talk to your doctor before taking any supplements, as they may interact with other medications or have side effects.

It's also important to note that while diet and nutrition can play a significant role in joint health, they are not the only factors to consider. Other lifestyle factors, such as exercise, stress management, and getting enough sleep, are also important for overall health and joint health.

In conclusion, maintaining a healthy diet is essential for joint health. Consuming a diet rich in fruits, vegetables, whole grains, lean proteins, and fatty fish can help reduce inflammation in the body and ease joint pain. Avoiding processed foods, red meat, fried foods, sugary beverages, and alcohol can also help maintain healthy joints. Incorporating healthy eating habits into your daily routine can help keep your joints healthy and pain-free. Additionally, staying hydrated, maintaining a healthy weight, limiting salt intake, and considering supplements may also contribute to optimal joint health. As always, it's important to talk to your doctor before making any significant changes to your diet or lifestyle.

Chapter ten:
Supplements for Joint Pain Relief: What Works and What Doesn't

Joint pain can be a debilitating condition that affects people of all ages. Whether it is caused by an injury, overuse, or a chronic condition such as arthritis, joint pain can limit mobility, reduce the quality of life, and lead to a cascade of health problems. For many people, supplements have become a popular way to manage joint pain, with a wide variety of options available on the market. But how do you know which supplements work, and which ones are just hype? In this chapter, we will explore the most commonly used supplements for joint pain relief, examining the scientific evidence behind each one.

Glucosamine and Chondroitin

Glucosamine and chondroitin are two supplements that are often marketed together for joint pain relief. Glucosamine is a natural substance found in cartilage, while chondroitin is a molecule that helps give cartilage its elasticity. Together, they are thought to help reduce inflammation, promote cartilage repair, and improve joint function.

So, do they work? The evidence is mixed. Some studies have shown that glucosamine and chondroitin can reduce joint pain and improve function, while others have found no significant benefit. One large study published in the New England Journal of Medicine found that the supplements were no more effective than placebo in reducing knee pain from osteoarthritis. Another meta-analysis of multiple studies found that the supplements were effective, but only for a subgroup of people with moderate to severe osteoarthritis.

Overall, if you are considering taking glucosamine and chondroitin for joint pain, it may be worth trying for a few months to see if you notice any improvement. However, keep in mind that the evidence is not definitive, and individual results may vary.

Omega-3 Fatty Acids

Omega-3 fatty acids are a type of healthy fat that is found in fish, nuts, and seeds. They are known to have anti-inflammatory properties, which may make them beneficial for reducing joint pain and stiffness.

The evidence for omega-3s and joint pain is somewhat mixed. Some studies have shown that taking omega-3 supplements can reduce inflammation and improve joint function, particularly in people with rheumatoid arthritis. However, other studies have found no significant benefit.

Even if omega-3s do not directly improve joint pain, they have many other health benefits, such as reducing inflammation throughout the body, promoting heart health, and supporting brain function. Therefore, it may be worth considering adding omega-3-rich foods or supplements to your diet for overall health.

Turmeric

Turmeric is a bright yellow spice that is commonly used in Indian and Middle Eastern cuisine. It contains a compound called curcumin, which has been shown to have anti-inflammatory properties.

Studies have found that curcumin may be beneficial for reducing joint pain and stiffness, particularly in people with osteoarthritis. One randomized controlled trial found that taking a curcumin supplement reduced knee pain and improved mobility in people with osteoarthritis, and another study found that a combination of curcumin and Boswellia (an herb with anti-inflammatory properties) was more effective than a placebo at reducing knee pain.

Keep in mind that curcumin is not well-absorbed by the body on its own, so it is often combined with other compounds to improve its bioavailability. Additionally, some people may experience side effects such as digestive upset or allergic reactions when taking curcumin supplements.

Boswellia

Boswellia is an herb that has been used for thousands of years in traditional medicine for its anti-inflammatory properties. It is thought to work by inhibiting the production of inflammatory compounds in the body.

Studies have found that taking a Boswellia supplement may help reduce joint pain and improve mobility in people with osteoarthritis and rheumatoid arthritis. One randomized controlled trial found that taking a Boswellia supplement for 8 weeks resulted in significant improvements in pain, stiffness, and physical function in people with osteoarthritis.

However, it is important to note that Boswellia may interact with certain medications, such as blood-thinning drugs, and may cause side effects such as digestive upset and allergic reactions in some people.

MSM

MSM (methylsulfonylmethane) is a sulfur-containing compound that is found in some foods and supplements. It is thought to have anti-inflammatory properties and may help reduce joint pain and stiffness.

The evidence for MSM and joint pain relief is somewhat mixed. Some studies have shown that taking MSM supplements can reduce joint pain and improve physical function, particularly in people with osteoarthritis. However, other studies have found no significant benefit.

It is important to note that MSM may interact with certain medications and may cause side effects such as digestive upset, headache, and allergic reactions in some people.

Vitamin D

Vitamin D is an important nutrient that is essential for bone health. It helps the body absorb calcium and maintain healthy bones and muscles. Some studies have also suggested that vitamin D may have anti-inflammatory properties and may help reduce joint pain and stiffness.

The evidence for vitamin D and joint pain relief is somewhat mixed. Some studies have found that low levels of vitamin D are associated with an increased risk of osteoarthritis and rheumatoid arthritis, while others have found no significant association.

If you are considering taking a vitamin D supplement for joint pain relief, it is important to speak with your healthcare provider first to determine if you are deficient in vitamin D and to determine the appropriate dosage.

Conclusion

In addition to supplements, many other lifestyle changes can help manage joint pain, such as maintaining a healthy weight, exercising regularly, practicing good posture, and avoiding activities that exacerbate joint pain. By combining these strategies, you can help reduce joint pain and improve your overall quality of life. Additionally, it is important to speak with your healthcare provider before starting any new supplement to ensure that it is safe and appropriate for you. It is also important to note that supplements are not a substitute for medical treatment, and if you have persistent joint pain or mobility issues, it is important to consult with your healthcare provider to determine the underlying cause and appropriate treatment.

Furthermore, it is crucial to carefully research and choose high-quality supplements from reputable manufacturers. Not all supplements are created equal, and some may contain contaminants or ineffective ingredients.

In addition to the supplements mentioned above, several other natural remedies may help reduce joint pain and stiffness. These include:

Turmeric: Turmeric is a spice that contains the compound curcumin, which has anti-inflammatory properties. Some studies have found that taking a turmeric supplement or adding turmeric to your diet may help reduce joint pain and improve physical function in people with osteoarthritis and rheumatoid arthritis.

Ginger: Ginger is another spice that has anti-inflammatory properties and may help reduce joint pain and stiffness. Some studies have found that taking a ginger supplement or drinking ginger tea may be beneficial for people with osteoarthritis.

Omega-3 fatty acids: Omega-3 fatty acids are a type of healthy fat that is found in fatty fish, such as salmon and tuna, as well as in fish oil supplements. Some studies have found that omega-3 supplements may help reduce joint pain and stiffness, particularly in people with rheumatoid arthritis.

Acupuncture: Acupuncture is a traditional Chinese medicine technique that involves inserting thin needles into specific points on the body to stimulate healing. Some studies have found that acupuncture may be beneficial for reducing joint pain and improving physical function in people with osteoarthritis and rheumatoid arthritis.

In conclusion, while several supplements may be beneficial for reducing joint pain and stiffness, it is important to carefully research and choose high-quality supplements from reputable manufacturers. Additionally, it is crucial to maintain a healthy lifestyle and consult with your healthcare provider to determine the underlying cause of joint pain and determine the appropriate treatment plan.

Chapter Eleven:

Lifestyle Changes for Joint Pain Management: Exercise, Sleep, and Stress Reduction

Living with joint pain can be challenging, but there are lifestyle changes you can make to help manage your symptoms. These changes include regular exercise, getting enough sleep, and reducing stress levels. In this chapter, we will explore each of these lifestyle changes in detail and provide you with practical tips and techniques for incorporating them into your daily routine.

Exercise for Joint Pain Management

Regular exercise is one of the most effective ways to manage joint pain. Exercise helps to improve joint mobility, increase muscle strength, and reduce inflammation. It also helps to improve mood, reduce stress levels, and promote overall health and well-being.

However, it is essential to choose the right type of exercise for your condition. Low-impact exercises such as walking, swimming, and cycling are ideal for people with joint pain. These exercises are gentle on the joints, and they help to improve cardiovascular fitness and muscle strength.

Strength training exercises are also important for joint pain management. These exercises help to increase muscle strength, which can help to support and protect the joints. Resistance bands, free weights, and weight machines are all effective tools for strength training.

Stretching exercises can also be beneficial for joint pain management. Stretching helps to improve flexibility, which can help to reduce joint stiffness and improve mobility. Yoga, Pilates, and tai chi are all excellent forms of stretching exercises that can help to improve joint health and reduce pain.

When starting an exercise program, it is essential to start slowly and gradually increase the intensity and duration of your workouts. It is also important to listen to your body and stop any exercise that causes pain or discomfort. Working with a physical therapist or personal trainer can also help develop a safe and effective exercise program.

Sleep for Joint Pain Management
Getting enough sleep is also essential for joint pain management. Sleep helps to reduce inflammation, improve mood, and promote overall health and well-being. However, joint pain can make it challenging to get a good night's sleep.

To improve sleep quality, it is essential to establish good sleep habits. This includes going to bed and waking up at the same time each day, creating a comfortable sleep environment, and avoiding stimulants such as caffeine and alcohol before bedtime. It is also important to avoid electronic devices such as smartphones and tablets before bedtime, as blue light can interfere with sleep.

Relaxation techniques such as deep breathing, meditation, and progressive muscle relaxation can also help improve sleep quality. These techniques help to reduce stress levels, which can improve sleep quality and reduce pain.

Stress Reduction for Joint Pain Management
Stress can also worsen joint pain. When you are stressed, your body releases hormones that can increase inflammation and pain. Therefore, reducing stress levels is essential for joint pain management.

Many techniques can help to reduce stress levels, including meditation, deep breathing, yoga, and tai chi. These techniques help to calm the mind and reduce the body's stress response. They also help to promote relaxation and improve mood.

Other techniques for reducing stress levels include practicing mindfulness, spending time in nature, and engaging in activities that you enjoy. It is also important to establish a good work-life balance and to avoid overcommitting yourself to work or other activities.

Conclusion

Managing joint pain requires a comprehensive approach that includes lifestyle changes such as regular exercise, getting enough sleep, and reducing stress levels. By incorporating these lifestyle changes into your daily routine, you can help to reduce pain, improve mobility, and promote overall health and well-being. It is also essential to work with your healthcare provider to develop a personalized treatment plan that addresses your individual needs and goals. With the right treatment and lifestyle changes, it is possible to live a full and active life with joint pain.

In addition to the types of exercises mentioned earlier, other activities can help to manage joint pain. For instance, water aerobics and other water-based activities can be beneficial for people with joint pain. Water provides buoyancy, which reduces stress on the joints, and the resistance of the water can provide a low-impact workout.

Low-impact exercises such as cycling can also be done on a stationary bike, which reduces the impact on the joints. This is especially beneficial for people who experience joint pain when walking or running.

Another type of exercise that can be helpful for joint pain management is range-of-motion exercises. These exercises help to improve joint mobility and reduce stiffness. Range-of-motion exercises involve moving the joint through its full range of motion, such as bending and straightening the knee or rotating the shoulder.

It is important to note that exercise should not be done to the point of pain. Some discomfort is expected when starting a new exercise program or increasing the intensity of an existing program. However, pain that persists or worsens during or after exercise may be a sign that the activity is too intense or not appropriate for your condition.

Sleep for Joint Pain Management

In addition to the tips mentioned earlier, other strategies can help to improve sleep quality. One such strategy is cognitive-behavioral therapy for insomnia (CBT-I). CBT-I is a type of therapy that helps to identify and change negative thoughts and behaviors that may be contributing to sleep problems. This type of therapy can be done individually or in a group setting and is often done by a trained therapist.

Another strategy for improving sleep quality is to maintain a sleep diary. A sleep diary can help you to identify patterns in your sleep and identify factors that may be contributing to sleep problems. This information can then be used to develop a personalized sleep plan.

Stress Reduction for Joint Pain Management

In addition to the techniques mentioned earlier, other strategies can help to reduce stress levels. One such strategy is to practice relaxation techniques throughout the day. This can include taking deep breaths, stretching, or doing a short meditation or visualization exercise.

Another strategy is to practice positive self-talk. This involves identifying negative thoughts and replacing them with positive, encouraging thoughts. For example, instead of saying "I can't do this," say "I am capable of handling this challenge."

In addition, it is important to seek support from friends, family, or a support group. Talking to others who understand what you are going through can help reduce and improve your mood.

Conclusion

In conclusion, lifestyle changes such as regular exercise, getting enough sleep, and reducing stress levels can be effective in managing joint pain. It is important to choose the right type of exercise for your condition, establish good sleep habits, and practice stress reduction techniques throughout the day. By incorporating these lifestyle changes into your daily routine, you can help to reduce pain, improve mobility, and promote overall health and well-being. It is also important to work with your healthcare provider to develop a personalized treatment plan that addresses your individual needs and goals.

Chapter twelve:
Integrative Approaches to Joint Pain Management: Combining Natural and Conventional Medicine

Joint pain is a common condition that affects millions of people worldwide. It can be caused by a variety of factors, including injury, arthritis, and other chronic conditions. While conventional medicine offers a range of treatments for joint pain, many people are turning to natural remedies to manage their symptoms. In this chapter, we will explore the benefits of combining natural and conventional medicine in the management of joint pain.

The Conventional Approach to Joint Pain Management

Conventional medicine offers several treatments for joint pain, depending on the underlying cause. In cases of acute joint pain caused by injury, rest, ice, and pain relievers such as ibuprofen and acetaminophen may be recommended. For chronic joint pain caused by conditions such as arthritis, nonsteroidal anti-inflammatory drugs (NSAIDs) or corticosteroid injections may be prescribed.

In more severe cases of joint pain, joint replacement surgery may be recommended. While these treatments can be effective, they often come with side effects and risks, and may not address the underlying causes of the pain.

The Natural Approach to Joint Pain Management

Many natural remedies have been used for centuries to treat joint pain. These remedies include:

Exercise and Physical Therapy: Exercise and physical therapy can help strengthen the muscles and joints, improving flexibility and reducing pain.

Dietary Changes: Certain foods, such as those high in omega-3 fatty acids, can reduce inflammation and relieve joint pain.

Supplements: Supplements such as glucosamine and chondroitin can help reduce joint pain and improve joint function.

Herbal Remedies: Herbs such as turmeric, ginger, and devil's claw have anti-inflammatory properties and can be effective in reducing joint pain.

While natural remedies can be effective in managing joint pain, they may not be enough for more severe cases or may take longer to show results. This is where the integration of natural and conventional medicine can be beneficial.

Integrative Approaches to Joint Pain Management

Integrative medicine combines conventional and natural medicine to provide a holistic approach to healthcare. When it comes to joint pain management, integrative medicine offers several benefits:

Reduced Side Effects: By combining natural remedies with conventional treatments, the dosages of medications can be reduced, reducing the risk of side effects.

Improved Results: Integrating natural remedies with conventional treatments can improve the effectiveness of treatment and provide faster relief of symptoms.

Personalized Treatment: Integrative medicine offers personalized treatment plans that take into account the individual's unique needs and preferences.

Better Long-Term Outcomes: Integrative medicine focuses on addressing the underlying causes of the pain rather than just treating the symptoms, leading to better long-term outcomes.

Integrative approaches to joint pain management may include:

Exercise and Physical Therapy: Exercise and physical therapy can be integrated with conventional treatments to improve joint function and reduce pain.

Dietary Changes: Dietary changes can be integrated with conventional treatments to reduce inflammation and relieve joint pain.

Supplements: Supplements can be integrated with conventional treatments to reduce joint pain and improve joint function.

Herbal Remedies: Herbal remedies can be integrated with conventional treatments to reduce inflammation and relieve joint pain.

Mind-Body Techniques: Mind-body techniques such as meditation and yoga can be integrated with conventional treatments to reduce stress and improve overall well-being.

Specifically, integrative approaches to joint pain management involve collaborating with a team of healthcare professionals, including medical doctors, physical therapists, nutritionists, and alternative medicine practitioners, to create a personalized treatment plan that addresses the individual's unique needs.

In addition to the natural remedies mentioned earlier, integrative medicine may also incorporate modalities such as acupuncture, massage therapy, and chiropractic care to alleviate joint pain and improve joint function.

Acupuncture, for example, is effective in reducing pain and improving joint mobility in patients with osteoarthritis.

Massage therapy can help relax the muscles surrounding the affected joint and improve blood flow, reducing inflammation and promoting healing. Chiropractic care can also help improve joint function by manipulating the spine and joints to alleviate pressure and restore proper alignment.

It is important to note that while integrative approaches to joint pain management can be effective, it is crucial to consult with a healthcare professional before starting any new treatment regimen, especially if taking medications or undergoing conventional treatments such as surgery. Natural remedies and alternative medicine modalities may interact with conventional treatments or medications, and it is important to ensure that any new treatments are safe and effective for the individual.

In conclusion, integrative approaches to joint pain management offer a holistic and personalized approach to managing joint pain. By combining natural and conventional medicine, patients can achieve faster and more effective relief of joint pain while addressing the underlying causes of the pain. However, it is crucial to consult with a healthcare professional before starting any new treatment regimen to ensure that it is safe and effective for the individual.

Conclusion

In conclusion, "Natural Joint Pain Remedy" is a comprehensive guide that offers readers various natural solutions to alleviate joint pain. The book covers a range of topics, from exercises to diet changes to natural supplements, all of which are intended to provide relief from joint pain. The book emphasizes the importance of a healthy lifestyle and offers practical tips on how to achieve it. The natural remedies offered in the book are safe, effective, and easy to implement, making it a valuable resource for anyone looking to manage joint pain without relying on pharmaceutical drugs. Overall, "Natural Joint Pain Remedy" is a must-read for anyone suffering from joint pain and looking for natural remedies to improve their quality of life.